Liver Transplant for Beginners

A Step-by-Step Guide to Surgery, Recovery, Nutrition, and Long-Term Care

mf

copyright © 2025 Brandon Gilta

All rights reserved No part of this book may be reproduced, or stored in a retrieval system, or transmitted in any form or by any means, electronic, mechanical, photocopying, recording, or otherwise, without express written permission of the publisher.

Disclaimer

By reading this disclaimer, you are accepting the terms of the disclaimer in full. If you disagree with this disclaimer, please do not read the guide.

All of the content within this guide is provided for informational and educational purposes only, and should not be accepted as independent medical or other professional advice. The author is not a doctor, physician, nurse, mental health provider, or registered nutritionist/dietician. Therefore, using and reading this guide does not establish any form of a physician-patient relationship.

Always consult with a physician or another qualified health provider with any issues or questions you might have regarding any sort of medical condition. Do not ever disregard any qualified professional medical advice or delay seeking that advice because of anything you have read in this guide. The information in this guide is not intended to be any sort of medical advice and should not be used in lieu of any medical advice by a licensed and qualified medical professional.

The information in this guide has been compiled from a variety of known sources. However, the author cannot attest to or guarantee the accuracy of each source and thus should not be held liable for any errors or omissions.

You acknowledge that the publisher of this guide will not be held liable for any loss or damage of any kind incurred as a result of this guide or the reliance on any information provided within this guide. You acknowledge and agree that you assume all risk and responsibility for any action you undertake in response to the information in this guide.

Using this guide does not guarantee any particular result (e.g., weight loss or a cure). By reading this guide, you acknowledge that there are no guarantees to any specific outcome or results you can expect.

All product names, diet plans, or names used in this guide are for identification purposes only and are the property of their respective owners. The use of these names does not imply endorsement. All other trademarks cited herein are the property of their respective owners.

Where applicable, this guide is not intended to be a substitute for the original work of this diet plan and is, at most, a supplement to the original work for this diet plan and never a direct substitute. This guide is a personal expression of the facts of that diet plan.

Where applicable, persons shown in the cover images are stock photography models and the publisher has obtained the rights to use the images through license agreements with third-party stock image companies.

Table of Contents

Introduction	7
What Is a Liver Transplant?	9
Why Liver Transplants Are Needed	9
Basic Terms Explained	10
How Liver Disease Progresses	12
Common Causes of Liver Disease	13
Who Might Need a Transplant	16
Signs You May Need a Transplant	16
Common Liver Conditions that Lead to Transplants	18
When to Ask Your Doctor About Next Steps	20
Preparing for Surgery (For Patients and Caregivers)	22
What to Expect in Pre-Surgery Evaluations	22
Emotional Prep: Fear, Hope, and Stress	24
Caregiver Tips: Helping Someone You Love Prepare	25
Questions to Ask Your Transplant Team	26
Understanding the Surgery Process	29
What Happens on Surgery Day	29
The Role of the Surgical Team	31
How Long Surgery Takes and What's Involved	32
Explaining It to Children or Loved Ones	33
What Recovery Looks Like (Step-by-Step)	36
Day 1: The First 24 Hours in the ICU	36
Days 2–3: Transition Out of the ICU	39
Days 4–7: Building Strength	44
Days 8–14 (or Longer): Preparing for Discharge	48
Common Side Effects and How to Handle Them	52
When You Might Go Home	55
The Caregiver's Role After Discharge	57
Your First 30 Days Post-Transplant	62

Building New Routines	62
Medication Management: What You Need to Know	63
Signs Something May Be Wrong (and What to Do)	65
Setting Up a Safe and Supportive Home Environment	66
Nutrition & Lifestyle for Liver Health	**68**
What to Eat and Avoid Post-Transplant	68
Easy Meal Ideas and Grocery Tips	70
Staying Active Without Overdoing It	71
Importance of Sleep and Stress Management	72
Long-Term Wellness and Support	**74**
Follow-Up Appointments and Lab Tests	74
Staying on Track with Your Medication	75
How to Talk to Your Employer or Insurance	76
Joining Support Groups for Patients or Caregivers	78
Conclusion	**80**
FAQs	**83**
References and Helpful Links	**86**

Introduction

Facing a liver transplant can feel like stepping into the unknown. Whether you're the patient preparing for surgery or a caregiver offering support, it's natural to feel overwhelmed. This guide is here to help make the process clearer, less intimidating, and more manageable for everyone involved.

Liver transplants are life-changing procedures, offering patients the chance to regain their health and quality of life. But the road to recovery is a journey, and knowing what to expect can make it much smoother. This guide breaks everything down into easy-to-follow sections so that you and your loved ones can feel better prepared every step of the way.

In this guide, we will talk about the following:

- What Is a Liver Transplant?
- Who Might Need a Transplant
- Preparing for Surgery (For Patients and Caregivers)
- Understanding the Surgery Process
- What Recovery Looks Like (Step by Step)
- Your First 30 Days Post-Transplant

- Nutrition & Lifestyle for Liver Health
- Long-Term Wellness and Support

Keep reading to learn more about liver transplants and how to prepare yourself for this life-saving procedure. By the end of this guide, you will have a better understanding of what to expect during the liver transplant process and how to take care of yourself afterwards.

What Is a Liver Transplant?

Liver transplants are complex, life-saving surgeries designed to address severe liver damage or failure when no other treatment options are effective. To better understand why these surgeries are needed and how they work, let's break it all down.

Why Liver Transplants Are Needed

Your liver is one of the most important organs in your body. It performs over 500 vital functions, including filtering toxins from your blood, processing nutrients, and producing bile to help you digest food. Your liver is essential for staying healthy, and unlike some other organs, there's no machine or medical substitute that can fully replicate its functions.

When the liver becomes severely damaged or diseased, it can't perform these critical tasks effectively. This is where a liver transplant might play a crucial role. A transplant is needed when the liver is so damaged that it cannot recover or continue working on its own. Without it, the condition can become life-threatening.

There are several reasons why someone might need a liver transplant. Some of the most common include:

- *Chronic liver disease* (long-lasting damage to the liver, often caused by conditions like hepatitis or heavy alcohol use).
- *Acute liver failure* (when the liver suddenly stops working, sometimes due to poisoning, severe infection, or certain medications).
- *Congenital conditions* (birth defects or inherited diseases like biliary atresia that affect liver function).

A liver transplant can save lives and dramatically improve quality of life. For many patients, it's the only option when other treatments fail to help.

Basic Terms Explained

The world of liver transplants can seem confusing at first, with lots of medical terms and jargon. Here are the most important ones you'll hear and what they mean:

1. **Donor**: The donor is the person who provides the healthy liver for transplantation. There are two types of donors:
   - *Deceased donors*: Someone who has passed away and whose family has agreed to donate their organs.

- ***Living donors***: A living person, often a relative or close friend, who donates a portion of their liver. This works because the liver can regrow and repair itself, a unique property of this organ. For example, a living donor can donate about 60% of their liver, which will grow back to full size within a few weeks.
2. **Recipient**: The recipient is the person who needs the transplant and receives the donor liver. During surgery, the damaged liver is completely or partially removed and replaced with the donated liver. The goal is to restore the recipient's health by giving them a functioning liver.
3. **MELD Score (Model for End-Stage Liver Disease)**: The MELD score is a number doctors use to measure how severe a patient's liver disease is and how urgently they need a transplant. The score is calculated based on lab tests that check your kidney function, blood clotting, and more. Think of it as a priority list for the transplant waiting list. The higher the MELD score, the sicker the patient and the more urgent their need for a new liver.

Understanding these basic terms is key to navigating the liver transplant process with clarity. By knowing the roles of donors, recipients, and the importance of the MELD score, you can better grasp how decisions are made and what to expect.

How Liver Disease Progresses

Liver disease usually doesn't cause major symptoms right away. This is why people often don't realize they're sick until the damage is severe. Let's look at how liver disease can quietly progress from mild to life-threatening over time.

1. *Early Stages*: At the beginning, the liver is inflamed. This is your body's response to an injury or infection, such as hepatitis (a liver infection) or excessive alcohol use. You might not feel any symptoms in this stage, but the inflammation can cause cells in your liver to become damaged.
2. *Steatosis (Fatty Liver)*: Over time, fat may build up in the liver, a condition called fatty liver disease. This is common in people with obesity, diabetes, or those who drink a lot of alcohol. Fat buildup might not cause immediate problems, but if left unchecked, it can lead to more serious issues.
3. *Fibrosis (Scar Tissue Formation)*: If the liver remains inflamed for a long time, scar tissue starts to form, a stage known as fibrosis. Think of scar tissue as patches that prevent the liver from functioning as well as it should. Unlike healthy liver cells, scar tissue doesn't perform any vital tasks in the body. At this point, some patients may start to experience symptoms like fatigue, nausea, or swelling.

4. ***Cirrhosis (Advanced Scarring)***: When fibrosis becomes widespread, it turns into cirrhosis. With cirrhosis, the liver becomes so scarred that it struggles to do its job. The symptoms become more noticeable, including yellowing of the skin (jaundice), abdominal swelling (ascites), or confusion caused by toxins affecting the brain (hepatic encephalopathy).
5. ***Liver Failure***: Eventually, the liver can't function at all. This can be sudden, such as in the case of acute liver failure caused by viral infections or toxic substances like overdoses. However, for many people, it's the result of years of ongoing liver damage. At this stage, a liver transplant is often the only option for survival.

Liver disease can progress silently, often going unnoticed until significant damage has occurred. Early detection and lifestyle changes are crucial to preventing its progression and protecting liver health.

Common Causes of Liver Disease

The liver is a vital organ responsible for many important functions, including filtering blood and removing toxins, producing bile to aid in digestion, storing energy as glycogen, and metabolizing fats, carbohydrates, and proteins. It's also the only organ in the body that can regenerate itself if damaged.

However, excessive or prolonged damage to the liver can lead to various forms of liver disease. Some common causes include:

1. *Hepatitis B and C*: These viral infections attack the liver over time, causing long-term damage that can lead to cirrhosis or cancer.
2. *Alcohol-Related Liver Disease*: Heavy, long-term alcohol use can severely damage liver cells and lead to scarring.
3. *Non-Alcoholic Fatty Liver Disease (NAFLD)*: This condition is linked to obesity and diabetes. Even though it isn't caused by alcohol, it can lead to cirrhosis if untreated.
4. *Genetic Disorders*: Some people inherit conditions like hemochromatosis, which causes the body to accumulate too much iron, or Wilson's disease, where copper builds up in the liver.
5. *Liver Tumors*: Liver cancer or large non-cancerous tumors may damage the liver enough to require a transplant.

Understanding how liver disease progresses can help you or a loved one recognize when symptoms might signal the need to talk to a doctor about potential treatments, including transplantation. Remember, early detection and maintaining a healthy lifestyle can slow or even stop liver disease from worsening.

By grasping these basics, you've already taken a crucial first step in navigating liver transplantation with confidence.

Who Might Need a Transplant

Liver transplantation is often the last line of defense for individuals with severe liver disease. Knowing the signs, understanding the conditions that lead to transplants, and recognizing when to seek guidance from a doctor can make a huge difference in managing your health or supporting a loved one.

Signs You May Need a Transplant

Severe liver disease can cause symptoms that affect almost every part of the body. These symptoms develop as the liver begins to fail and struggles to perform its vital functions. Here's a closer look at some of the key warning signs:

- *Yellowing of the Skin or Eyes (Jaundice)*: Jaundice occurs when the liver can't process a substance called bilirubin, which builds up in the blood and turns the skin and eyes yellow. It's one of the clearest indicators that the liver is struggling.
- *Fluid Buildup in the Abdomen (Ascites)*: If the liver can't properly manage the body's fluid balance, excess fluid can collect in the abdomen. This often results in

swelling, discomfort, and a tight feeling in the stomach area.
- ***Confusion or Difficulty Thinking (Hepatic Encephalopathy)***: A failing liver may allow toxins, such as ammonia, to accumulate in the bloodstream. These toxins can travel to the brain and cause confusion, mood swings, forgetfulness, or even severe disorientation.
- ***Severe Fatigue and Weakness***: The liver plays a key role in your energy levels. When it's not functioning properly, it can leave you feeling exhausted, even after rest. This is often paired with muscle loss, since the liver isn't able to process nutrients efficiently.
- ***Bleeding or Easy Bruising***: The liver produces proteins needed for blood clotting. If it begins to fail, you might bruise easily or experience prolonged bleeding from minor injuries.
- ***Frequent and Severe Infections***: The liver helps manage your immune system. A weakened liver may make it harder for your body to fight off infections, leading to more frequent or longer-lasting illnesses.

If you or someone you care for is experiencing these symptoms, it's important to reach out to a doctor immediately. These may indicate serious liver damage that could require advanced treatment.

Common Liver Conditions that Lead to Transplants

Several health conditions can result in liver damage so severe that a transplant becomes necessary. Here's an overview of the most common ones:

1. **Cirrhosis (Severe Scarring of the Liver)**: Cirrhosis develops when prolonged liver damage causes scar tissue to replace healthy tissue. This limits the liver's ability to function. Cirrhosis has many causes, including chronic alcohol use, viral infections (hepatitis), and fatty liver disease. The signs of liver failure from cirrhosis typically include jaundice, fluid buildup, and confusion.
2. **Hepatitis B and C**: These viral infections cause chronic inflammation in the liver, leading to progressive damage over years or even decades. Hepatitis C is one of the leading causes of liver transplants globally, as it often leads to cirrhosis or liver cancer if untreated.
3. **Non-Alcoholic Fatty Liver Disease (NAFLD)**: NAFLD is common in people with obesity, diabetes, or metabolic syndrome. Over time, fat deposits in the liver can lead to inflammation, fibrosis, and cirrhosis, even in those who don't drink alcohol.
4. **Alcohol-Related Liver Disease (ARLD)**: Heavy drinking over many years can destroy healthy liver

tissue, often leading to cirrhosis. Abstaining from alcohol can sometimes reverse early liver damage, but advanced cases may still require a transplant.

5. **Acute Liver Failure**: Sometimes the liver fails suddenly. This can be caused by infections, drug toxicity (such as acetaminophen overdose), or autoimmune diseases. Unlike chronic conditions, acute liver failure progresses very quickly and is often life-threatening without intervention.

6. **Liver Cancer**: Certain cancers that begin in the liver, like hepatocellular carcinoma (HCC), can sometimes be treated with surgery. However, if the cancer is extensive but hasn't spread beyond the liver, a transplant may still be an option.

7. **Other Rare Conditions**:
   - *Autoimmune Hepatitis*: The immune system mistakenly attacks the liver, causing long-term inflammation and damage.
   - *Wilson's Disease*: A rare genetic disorder where copper builds up in the liver.
   - *Hemochromatosis*: A condition where excessive iron accumulates in the liver, leading to damage.

These common liver conditions highlight the critical role the liver plays in overall health and how severe damage can lead to the need for a transplant. Early detection and proper management are key to preventing progression and ensuring better outcomes.

When to Ask Your Doctor About Next Steps

Recognizing when it's time to talk to your doctor about liver transplantation can be challenging. However, there are clear signs that should prompt a serious conversation:

- *Worsening Symptoms*: If jaundice, fluid buildup, or mental confusion are getting worse despite medical care, it's time to ask if transplantation might be necessary.
- *Frequent Hospital Stays*: Patients who find themselves repeatedly hospitalized due to liver-related complications (like fluid drainage or infections) may be reaching the point where a transplant is needed.
- *Mention of MELD Score*: If your doctor starts discussing your MELD score, this means they're tracking how advanced your liver disease is. A high MELD score is a strong indicator to start exploring transplant options.

Preparing for a conversation about transplantation can feel overwhelming, but it's an important step. Here are some tips to make it easier:

1. **Write Down Questions Beforehand**: Some useful questions to ask include:

- What stage is my liver disease, and how urgent is my condition?
- Am I a candidate for a transplant, and what steps are involved in getting on a transplant list?
- Are there alternative treatments I should try first?

2. **<u>Bring a Caregiver or Family Member</u>**: Having someone with you can help you remember information, write notes, and provide emotional support.
3. **<u>Be Honest About Symptoms</u>**: Tell your doctor about all the symptoms you've been experiencing, no matter how small they seem. Even mild symptoms can provide critical information about your liver health.
4. **<u>Ask About Next Steps</u>**: If a transplant seems probable, ask your doctor what comes next. This usually involves a referral to a transplant center for more specialized evaluations.

By staying proactive and open with your healthcare team, you can ensure you're taking the right steps to manage your liver condition and explore all available treatment options, including transplantation. Remember, you don't have to face this process alone—your doctor, family, and support networks are there to help.

Preparing for Surgery (For Patients and Caregivers)

Preparing for a liver transplant involves more than just medical tests; it's also a mental and emotional process. Whether you're the patient or the caregiver, understanding what lies ahead can make the experience less daunting.

This chapter will walk you through everything from pre-surgery evaluations to managing emotions and practical tips for caregivers.

What to Expect in Pre-Surgery Evaluations

Before being approved for a liver transplant, patients undergo an extensive medical and psychological evaluation. This ensures that the surgery is the best option and that your body is ready for the procedure.

1. ***Blood Tests***: Blood tests help determine your overall health and how well your liver is functioning. They measure things like your kidney function, blood clotting ability, and whether you have any infections.

2. ***Imaging Scans (Ultrasound, CT, or MRI)***: These scans are used to get a detailed look at your liver and surrounding areas. They help doctors assess the extent of damage and check for any complications, such as tumors or blockages in blood flow.
3. ***Heart and Lung Tests***: Since liver transplantation is a major surgery, your heart and lungs must be strong enough to handle it. Tests like an electrocardiogram (EKG) or chest X-ray will assess how well these vital organs are functioning.
4. ***Psychological Assessment***: Transplants are as demanding emotionally as they are physically. A psychologist or counselor may evaluate your emotional readiness and ability to follow the lifelong care plan required after surgery.
5. ***Nutrition Check with a Dietitian***: Malnutrition can affect recovery, so a dietitian will assess your current diet and recommend changes. Sometimes, patients need to gain or lose weight before surgery.
6. ***Meeting the Transplant Team***: You'll speak with various specialists, including surgeons, hepatologists (liver specialists), and transplant coordinators. Each member of the team plays a critical role in your care, from surgery preparation to aftercare. Think of this as your chance to ask questions and establish a trusting relationship with the team who will guide you through the process.

These pre-surgery evaluations are crucial to ensure you're physically and mentally prepared for a liver transplant. By working closely with your transplant team, you'll be set up for the best possible outcome.

Emotional Prep: Fear, Hope, and Stress

Undergoing a liver transplant comes with a mix of emotions, including fear, hope, and uncertainty. Here's how to prepare emotionally for the road ahead:

1. ***Acknowledge Your Feelings***: It's normal to feel scared or anxious. Surgery is a big step, and uncertainty about the future can be overwhelming. Talk about your feelings with someone you trust, whether it's a loved one, therapist, or support group. Bottling up emotions can make anxiety worse.
2. ***Find Hope Amid Fear***: Remind yourself why you're taking this step. A liver transplant offers the opportunity for a healthier, longer life. Focus on the positives, like enjoying more time with loved ones or resuming activities you've had to put on hold.
3. *Coping with Stress*
   - *Mindfulness Exercises*: Deep breathing, journaling, or guided meditations can help you stay calm.

- *Join a Support Group*: Talking with others who've gone through a transplant can help you feel less alone.
- *Set Small Goals*: Instead of worrying about the entire process, focus on one step at a time, such as completing evaluations or packing for your hospital stay.

Try to lean on your support system. Family and friends can provide both emotional comfort and help with practical tasks, so you don't feel like you're carrying all the weight alone.

Caregiver Tips: Helping Someone You Love Prepare

If you're a caregiver, your role in this process is invaluable. Preparing someone you love for a transplant is about more than logistical help; it's about being their anchor during this life-changing time.

1. **Provide Emotional Support**: Be a good listener. Patients may feel scared or guilty about the burden the transplant process can place on others. Reassure them that you're there to help and remind them it's okay to feel the way they do.
2. **Stay Organized**
    - *Log Important Information*: Keep track of medical appointments, test results, and contact

names for the transplant team. A notebook or digital app can make this easier.
   - *Help with Paperwork*: Filling out forms for insurance companies or financial aid programs can feel overwhelming for someone who's already stressed. Offer to assist with these tasks.
3. **Plan for the Hospital Stay**: Pack a bag with essentials like clothing, toiletries, medications, and items that will bring comfort, such as books or a favorite blanket.
4. **Look After Yourself**: Caregiving can take a physical and emotional toll. Stay healthy by eating balanced meals, getting enough rest, and taking regular breaks. Don't hesitate to lean on your own support system or join caregiver support groups.

Remember, you can't pour from an empty cup. Taking care of yourself allows you to better care for your loved one.

Questions to Ask Your Transplant Team

Knowledge is power, and understanding the process helps reduce anxiety for both patients and caregivers. Here are some important questions to ask your transplant team during your consultations:

1. **About the Procedure:**
   - How long will the surgery take?
   - What are the risks and success rates?

- Will the new liver come from a living or deceased donor?

2. **Preparing for Surgery:**
   - Are there lifestyle changes or medications I need to follow before the transplant?
   - How long will I be in the hospital?

3. **After Surgery:**
   - What can I expect during recovery?
   - Will I need physical therapy or rehab?
   - How soon can I return to daily activities like work or exercise?

4. **Medications and Follow-Up Care:**
   - What types of medications will I need to take?
   - How often will I need follow-up appointments and lab tests?

5. **Advice for Caregivers:**
   - How can caregivers best support a loved one recovering from transplant surgery?
   - Are there specific signs caregivers should watch for during recovery?

Your transplant team is there to ensure you feel informed and confident. Don't be afraid to ask for clarifications or raise concerns; they are your partners in this journey.

Preparing for a liver transplant involves more than just surgery; it requires teamwork, planning, and emotional support. By understanding what's ahead and using this time to create a strong foundation, you'll be better equipped to face surgery day with courage and hope.

Understanding the Surgery Process

The day of a liver transplant is a significant milestone in the patient's medical journey. Knowing what to expect can help ease fears and make the process feel more manageable for both patients and their loved ones. This chapter provides an overview of the events, people, and steps involved in the surgery process.

What Happens on Surgery Day

On the day of surgery, there's a lot to prepare and manage, but the hospital staff will guide you every step of the way. Here's a breakdown of how the day unfolds:

1. *Arrival at the Hospital*: You'll be asked to check in several hours before the surgery begins. This allows plenty of time for final preparations. Once you arrive, you'll be directed to the pre-surgery area.
2. *Pre-Surgery Preparations*:

- *Vital Signs Check*: Nurses will measure your heart rate, blood pressure, and temperature to ensure everything is stable.
- *IV Line Placement*: A nurse will place an intravenous (IV) line in your arm to deliver fluids and medications during surgery.
- *Meeting Your Team*: The anesthesiologist and surgeon will review the procedure with you, answer any last-minute questions, and make sure you're comfortable.
- *Consent Forms*: You or your legal representative may need to sign forms to confirm your understanding of the surgery.
- *Final Instructions*: You'll be asked to change into a hospital gown, remove any jewelry, and follow any other specific pre-surgery instructions.

3. ***Heading to the Operating Room (OR)***: When everything is ready, you'll be taken to the OR. Caregivers can usually wait in a designated area where the surgical team will give updates as the surgery progresses.
4. ***Anesthesia Administration***: The anesthesiologist will administer general anesthesia, ensuring you're completely unconscious and pain-free during the procedure.

The day of surgery may feel overwhelming, but the hospital team ensures everything is well-coordinated and you're supported at every step. By understanding the process, you can feel more prepared and confident as you head into surgery.

The Role of the Surgical Team

A liver transplant surgery involves a highly skilled team of medical professionals, each playing a specific role to ensure the procedure's success. Here's a look at some of the key players:

- ***Transplant Surgeon***: The lead doctor who performs the surgery. The surgeon is responsible for removing the damaged liver and attaching the new one with precise care.
- ***Anesthesiologist***: This specialist monitors your breathing, heart rate, and other vital signs while managing your anesthesia. They ensure you're safe and comfortable throughout the operation.
- ***Surgical Nurses***: Nurses work alongside the surgeon to assist with instruments, maintain a sterile environment, and respond to any surgical needs.
- ***Perfusionist (if applicable)***: Sometimes, during complex procedures, a perfusionist manages equipment that temporarily takes over the functions of the heart and lungs.

- ***Transplant Coordinator***: Although not in the operating room, the transplant coordinator ensures everyone involved is updated on the process. They also guide caregivers on where to go and what to expect.

The entire team works together seamlessly to handle any challenges that may arise and to give the patient the best possible care.

How Long Surgery Takes and What's Involved

Liver transplant surgery is a long and intricate procedure. Here's a simple breakdown of what's involved:

1. ***Anesthesia***: The patient is placed under general anesthesia, meaning they'll stay asleep for the entire surgery.
2. ***Incision and Access***: The surgeon makes an incision in the abdomen to access the liver. The size and location of the incision depend on your specific condition and whether the liver comes from a deceased or living donor.
3. ***Removing the Damaged Liver***: The surgeon carefully detaches the diseased liver from surrounding veins and blood vessels. This step must be done meticulously to avoid complications.
4. ***Attaching the Donor Liver***: The donor liver is brought into the operating room, where the surgeon attaches it

to the patient's blood vessels and bile ducts. This allows blood and bile to flow properly through the transplanted liver.
5. *Checking for Function and Closing the Incision*: Before finishing, the surgeon ensures that the new liver is functioning properly and that bleeding is controlled. The incision is then closed with sutures or staples.

Duration: A liver transplant typically takes between 6 and 12 hours. The complexity of the surgery, the patient's condition, and any complications can affect the total time.

Explaining It to Children or Loved Ones

Patients undergoing transplant surgery often have children or loved ones who are anxious or unsure about the process. Here's how to explain it in a reassuring and age-appropriate way:

For Children:
1. *Use Simple Language*: "The doctors are going to fix my liver so that it works better. Right now, it's not doing its job well, and this surgery will help me get healthier."
2. *Focus on Positives*: Explain that the transplant will help you feel stronger and give you more energy to do things with them.
3. *Answer Their Questions Honestly*: Kids may ask things like, "Will it hurt?" or "Will you be okay?" You

can answer by saying, "The doctors will make sure I'm comfortable, and they're going to take very good care of me."
4. **Reassure Them**: Remind them that there will be people to take care of them while you're in the hospital, and they can visit or talk to you often.

For Other Family Members:
1. **Share Basic Information**: Explain the steps of the surgery in simple terms. For example, you might say, "The surgeons will replace my liver with a healthy one and make sure it's working properly during the surgery."
2. **Address Concerns**: Family members may worry about the risks. It's okay to acknowledge these risks while emphasizing that the transplant team is experienced and well-prepared.
3. **Provide Updates**: Designate someone to share updates with loved ones during the surgery, especially if it's a long procedure.
4. **Encourage Support**: Ask loved ones to lean on each other, as emotional support can help everyone cope during this time.

By understanding the surgery process and communicating openly, both patients and their families can feel more prepared and supported. While surgery day may feel overwhelming, it's a crucial step toward better health and a brighter future.

What Recovery Looks Like (Step-by-Step)

Recovering from a liver transplant is a gradual process that requires patience, teamwork, and ongoing care. While everyone's experience is unique, this chapter will give you a step-by-step guide to what recovery might look like—from your time in the hospital to the important role caregivers play after discharge.

After surgery, patients typically remain in the hospital for 1 to 2 weeks to ensure the new liver is functioning well and there are no major complications. Here's what you can expect:

Day 1: The First 24 Hours in the ICU

The first day after your liver transplant is a critical time for your body to adjust to the new organ, and your medical team will take every precaution to make sure you're safe and comfortable. After the surgery, you will wake up in the Intensive Care Unit (ICU), where nursing staff and doctors can monitor you closely. This can feel overwhelming at first, but it's all part of helping your body heal properly.

What to Expect in the ICU

1. **Monitoring Your Health:**

   When you wake up, you'll notice that you're attached to several medical devices. This might feel strange, but these are vital for monitoring how your body is adjusting to the new liver. Here's what you can expect:

   - *IV Lines*: These thin tubes in your arms or neck deliver important fluids and medications, including pain medications and anti-rejection drugs.
   - *Drains*: Surgical drains may be placed near your incision to remove any excess fluid from the surgery area. This helps prevent infections and promotes healing.
   - *Catheter*: A urinary catheter will collect your urine to help the team monitor your kidney health and hydration levels.

   Although this equipment might seem intimidating, it's all standard in post-transplant care and ensures your recovery is progressing smoothly.

2. **Pain Management:**

   After surgery, it's normal to feel some soreness or pressure around your incision site. Many patients also feel tightness or stiffness in their abdomen. Don't worry, the medical team will keep a close eye on your pain levels and provide medication to keep you as comfortable as possible. If you're feeling any discomfort, be sure to tell the nurses so they can adjust your pain relief accordingly.

3. **Ventilator Support:**

   When you wake up, you may have a breathing tube in your mouth connected to a ventilator. This helps your body get enough oxygen while the effects of anesthesia are still wearing off. The ventilator is only a temporary measure and will be removed as soon as you're strong enough to breathe on your own.

For most people, this happens within the first day. If the breathing tube is still in place when you wake up, know that it's a normal part of the recovery process, and the team will explain everything to help you feel at ease.

4. **Rest and Recovery:**

   On this first day, your job is to rest. Your body has been through a major operation, and the medical team wants you to conserve your energy. You won't be getting out of bed just yet, but nurses may encourage light movements like wiggling your toes or shifting positions to keep your blood circulating.

For Caregivers

While caregivers play a big role in the recovery process, access to the ICU is often limited. This helps the medical team focus on giving the patient around-the-clock care during this critical phase. Caregivers might not be able to see you right away, but the team will give them frequent updates about your progress. Encourage your family or caregiver to rest during this time, as the days ahead may require more involvement.

It's natural to feel nervous or unsure during this time, but you're in the best possible hands. The ICU staff is experienced in caring for transplant patients and is there to answer your questions and make you as comfortable as possible. Every machine and every step is designed to help your body recover safely and quickly.

Days 2–3: Transition Out of the ICU

The second and third days after your liver transplant mark an exciting and important step in your recovery. These are the days when your body begins to stabilize, and you'll notice progress toward regaining independence.

During this phase, the medical team will focus on helping you get stronger, ensuring your new liver is functioning well, and introducing you to the medications that will help protect your transplant for life.

Moving to a Regular Hospital Room

If your condition remains stable after the first 24 hours, you'll move from the Intensive Care Unit (ICU) to a regular hospital room. This transition shows that your body is adjusting well to the new liver and no longer needs constant intensive monitoring. The environment in a regular hospital room is quieter and more private, which can help you rest better and begin focusing on recovery.

Here's what moving to the regular room might feel like:

- You will still have some medical devices, such as IV lines or surgical drains, but you'll gradually rely on them less.
- Nurses will still monitor your vitals and liver function closely, but the team will now encourage you to become more involved in your own care.
- Caregivers may have easier access to visit you, allowing them to become more involved in your recovery.

A regular hospital room is an encouraging milestone that signals your progress.

Starting Light Physical Activity

Two key goals during this stage are to help you strengthen your body and reduce the risk of complications, like blood clots or lung issues. To do this, the medical team will guide you through small movements and exercises designed to keep your body active without pushing it too hard.

Here's what you'll work on:

1. ***Getting Out of Bed***: Nurses will help you sit up in bed and move to a chair for short periods. Over time, you'll take a few steps with assistance, such as walking across the room or down the hall.
2. ***Brief Walks***: While these may feel tiring at first, short walks are vital for improving circulation and boosting your strength. Even a few slow steps are considered a big win.
3. ***Shallow Breathing Exercises***: You'll be encouraged to do light respiratory exercises to strengthen your lungs and prevent pneumonia. Often, patients use a tool called an incentive spirometer, which helps you practice taking deep breaths. It may feel strange at first, but these exercises are important to keep your lungs healthy.

Your medical team understands you may feel weak or unsteady during these initial steps. Remember that no movement is too small, and every step is part of the healing process.

Introduction to Anti-Rejection Medications

Starting on Day 2, you'll be introduced to anti-rejection medications, also called immunosuppressants. These medications play a critical role in protecting your new liver by preventing your immune system from recognizing it as foreign and attacking it.

Here's what you need to know about these medications during this phase:

- ***Why They're Important***: Your immune system is naturally designed to protect you from anything it views as unfamiliar, such as viruses or bacteria. Since your new liver comes from a donor, your body may see it as foreign. Anti-rejection medications help "teach" your immune system to accept the new liver.
- ***Types of Medications***: The transplant team will likely prescribe several kinds of immunosuppressants, alongside other medications to prevent infections or manage side effects.
- ***Lifelong Commitment***: These drugs are essential for the rest of your life. The medical team will explain their purpose and teach you how to take them correctly.

This is a good time to ask questions and start learning more about your medication regimen. Don't feel shy about asking the nurses or pharmacy staff about side effects or tips for staying on schedule. They're there to support you.

What You Might Feel

It's perfectly normal to feel a range of emotions during this transition—from relief and excitement to fatigue and unease. You've already come so far, and though these first steps may feel small, they're incredibly meaningful. You may also feel tired or overwhelmed as your body adjusts to even light activity. Be patient with yourself and celebrate any progress, no matter how minor.

<u>Tips for Caregivers</u>

- Encourage the patient to take small steps, literally and figuratively. Offer positive reinforcement for every effort, even sitting up in bed or completing one respiratory exercise.
- Watch and learn from the medical team, especially when it comes to exercises or medication instructions. This will prepare you to provide effective support at home.
- Be present. Your encouragement and emotional support mean a lot during this phase.

By the end of Days 2–3, you'll be more active and independent, and you'll have started getting used to your new medication routine. This phase sets the stage for the next steps in your recovery, including building strength and gaining more independence. With your medical team and caregivers by your side, you're on a steady path toward healing and returning home.

Days 4–7: Building Strength

During Days 4 through 7 of your recovery, the focus shifts toward rebuilding strength and helping your body continue to heal. You'll notice your activity level increasing bit by bit and start feeling more like yourself.

This phase is all about baby steps that lead to big progress. The medical team will guide you as you work on regaining physical strength and transitioning your diet to be more nourishing and supportive for your recovering body.

Increasing Physical Activity

By this stage, staying active becomes a key part of your recovery. Moving around helps improve blood circulation, prevent complications like blood clots, and build up your overall stamina. Even though it may feel tough at first, these small exercises are crucial for regaining your strength.

Here's what you can expect for physical activity during this phase:

- *More Frequent Movement*: Nurses and physical therapists will encourage you to get out of bed more often, whether it's sitting in a chair or taking brief walks in the hallway. They'll support and guide you every step of the way.
- *Building Stamina*: Your walks will gradually increase in distance and duration. These short strolls help

improve circulation, which speeds up your body's healing process.
- *Light Exercises*: Physical therapists might introduce gentle exercises or stretches tailored to your abilities. These movements focus on building flexibility and strength without straining your body.
- *Rest Periods*: While movement is essential, rest is just as important. You'll alternate between activity and rest to ensure your body doesn't get overly tired.

It's perfectly normal to feel tired or sore as you begin to increase your activity levels. Progress might feel slow, but every small achievement, like taking a few steps further than the day before, is a sign that you're headed in the right direction.

Transitioning Your Diet

Your digestive system begins to recover during this phase, which means you'll start eating a wider variety of foods. It's an exciting step because nourishing your body with the right foods is important for healing and energy.

Here's what the diet transition typically looks like:

- *From Liquids to Solids*: Early in your recovery, you might have been on a limited liquid diet. Now, the medical team will gradually introduce soft, easy-to-digest foods, such as mashed potatoes, oatmeal, or soups. Over time, you'll progress to small portions of solid foods.

- **Balanced Nutrition**: A diet following a transplant emphasizes nutritious, well-rounded meals made up of lean proteins, fresh fruits, vegetables, whole grains, and healthy fats. This approach ensures your body gets the essential nutrients required for recovery and healing.
- **Hydration**: Drinking enough fluids remains critical. You'll be encouraged to take small sips throughout the day if your fluid intake is restricted. Keeping hydrated helps your body function properly and supports liver health.
- **Avoiding Certain Foods**: There may be dietary restrictions to protect your new liver. Examples include avoiding raw or undercooked foods, high-sodium meals, or foods that could interfere with your medications. Your dietitian will guide you on what's safe to eat.

If you have trouble eating or feel nauseous, share your concerns with the team. They can adjust your meal plan to make things easier for you.

Building Confidence and Independence

As you become more physically active and adjust to eating regular meals, you'll also start regaining a sense of independence. You'll find yourself able to do small tasks like grooming or sitting up on your own for longer periods. The medical team will continue to supervise your progress and make sure everything is on track.

What You Might Feel

It's important to remember that everyone's recovery looks different. Some days, you might feel energetic and ready to move around, while other days might feel more tiring. This is entirely normal. You're still in the early stages of healing, and your body is doing a lot of hard work behind the scenes. Celebrate every small accomplishment, whether it's taking an extra lap around the hall or finishing your meal.

Tips for Caregivers

- *Cheer on Progress*: Encourage the patient to take small steps in physical activity and try new foods, even if they still feel unsure. Positive reinforcement goes a long way.
- *Learn Together*: Caregivers can work alongside the medical team to understand the importance of movement and dietary adjustments. This will help when it's time to transition home.
- *Be Patient*: Recovery varies from person to person, so it's essential to maintain a compassionate and understanding approach when progress feels slow.

By the end of Days 4–7, you'll likely feel more mobile and comfortable with your new diet. These days are important for building a strong foundation as you prepare for the next stage of your recovery. Keep focusing on the small wins, trust the guidance of your medical team, and rely on your support system as you move forward.

Days 8–14 (or Longer): Preparing for Discharge

By Days 8–14, you'll likely feel stronger and more confident in your recovery. This phase marks a turning point as the focus shifts from hospital-based care to getting ready for life at home.

The medical team will work closely with you and your caregiver to ensure you're prepared to manage your recovery safely and effectively. While it's natural to feel a mix of emotions about going home, the team will arm you with the knowledge and tools you need for success.

Discharge Education

Discharge planning is an important part of this phase. The medical staff will spend time teaching you and your caregiver how to take care of yourself once you leave the hospital. They'll cover several key topics:

1. *Wound Care*:
    - You'll be shown how to care for the incision site to keep it clean and promote healing. This

might include learning how to change dressings and what types of products are safe to use.
- The nurses will point out what to watch for, such as redness, swelling, or drainage, which could indicate an infection. If you notice anything unusual, report it to your medical team right away.
2. ***Recognizing Signs of Complications***: Staying alert to any warning signs of complications is crucial during recovery. The medical staff will explain what symptoms to keep an eye on, such as:
    - Fever, chills, or sweats, which could signal an infection.
    - Jaundice (yellowing of the skin), which might indicate a liver issue.
    - Sudden pain or swelling near the incision site or legs, which could indicate complications like a clot or infection.
    - Knowing when to call your doctor or seek medical help will give you and your caregiver peace of mind.
3. ***Medication Schedule***: By this point, you'll already be taking your anti-rejection medications and other prescriptions, but the medical team will focus on making sure you're comfortable managing them independently:

- You'll learn the correct doses, times, and any dietary or lifestyle considerations tied to your medications.
- The team may provide a chart, pill organizer, or reminders to help you stay on track.
- They'll discuss side effects, what's normal, and when to contact your doctor.
- Medications will be a long-term part of your life, and understanding their importance now can set you up for success outside the hospital.

4. ***Diet and Activity Guidance***: The staff will ensure you're following a post-transplant diet plan that promotes healing and maintains liver health. This includes avoiding harmful foods and prioritizing balanced meals. Alongside dietary advice, they'll also guide you on safe levels of physical activity to continue improving your strength at home.

Follow-Up Appointments

Your recovery doesn't end when you leave the hospital. Regular follow-up care is critical, especially in the first weeks post-surgery. Before discharge, you'll be provided with a schedule for these checkups:

- *Frequent Visits*: At the beginning, follow-up visits might be weekly or even more frequent, depending on your condition. During these visits, doctors will

monitor your liver function, medication levels, and overall recovery.
- ***Blood Tests***: You'll likely need regular blood work to check how well the liver is working and ensure the medications are doing their job without causing side effects.
- ***Adjustments***: Medications might be adjusted based on your test results, so it's important to attend every appointment and ask any questions about your progress.

What You Might Be Feeling

This stage can bring a mix of feelings. You might be excited to leave the hospital but also nervous about managing your recovery at home. These emotions are completely normal. Remember, you're not alone in this process. The medical team will be there to answer questions, and regular follow-ups will provide ongoing support.

Physically, you might still feel tired or weaker than usual, but this is a natural part of healing. Go at your own pace and give yourself time to regain strength.

Tips for Caregivers

- ***Pay Attention During Education***: Caregivers play a key role in making the transition home smoother. Attend all discharge education sessions and take notes if necessary.

- **Support Medication Management**: Help create a tracking system for medications to ensure consistent dosing.
- **Be Encouraging**: Recovery can feel overwhelming for the patient, so offer positive reinforcement and assist with daily tasks as they rebuild independence.
- **Know When to Seek Help**: Familiarize yourself with the signs of complications so you can act quickly if needed.

By the time you're discharged, you'll have a solid plan in place to manage your recovery at home. These preparations set you up for a safe transition and continued progress. Remember, recovery is a step-by-step process, and both you and your caregiver are supported by an experienced medical team every step of the way. Soon, you'll be taking even more steps toward returning to your normal activities and enjoying life with your new liver!

Common Side Effects and How to Handle Them

It's normal to experience some side effects after a liver transplant as your body heals and adjusts to the new organ. Here are some common ones and simple ways to manage them:

1. **Pain at the Incision Site**: You might feel soreness or tightness around the area where the surgery was done.

What You Can Do:

- Take the pain medications your doctor prescribed to stay comfortable.
- Avoid lifting heavy objects or doing activities that put strain on your abdomen until you're cleared by your medical team.

2. *Fatigue*: Feeling tired is very common after such a big surgery. Recovery takes time, and it's normal to feel low on energy for weeks or even months.

What You Can Do:

- Give yourself plenty of rest and take breaks often.
- Balance light activity with downtime.
- Eating healthy meals and drinking plenty of fluids can help you gain energy over time.

3. *Swelling (Edema)*: Your legs or feet might swell because of fluid buildup after surgery.

What You Can Do:

- When you sit, elevate your legs to help reduce the swelling.
- Wearing compression socks may help if your doctor recommends them.
- Try to walk as much as you're able to, as light activity can improve circulation and reduce swelling.

4. ***Nausea or Digestive Issues***: The medications that protect your new liver might upset your stomach or change your appetite. Diarrhea or nausea can also happen.

What You Can Do:

- Take your medicine with food to make it easier on your stomach.
- If big meals make you feel sick, try eating smaller amounts more frequently.
- Talk to your doctor if these issues persist, as they may adjust your medications or offer other solutions.

5. ***Risk of Infection***: Your immune system is weaker because of the medications that help prevent rejection of your new liver. This means even small infections can become serious.

What You Can Do:

- Wash your hands often and keep your living space clean.
- Be careful during flu season or avoid crowded areas if possible.
- If you feel feverish, have chills, or notice flu-like symptoms, contact your doctor immediately.

When to Call the Team

If you're unsure whether something you're feeling is normal, reach out to your transplant team right away. Quick action can help stop small problems before they become serious.

You're not alone in this process, and your medical team is there to guide and support you throughout your recovery. Take it one step at a time, and remember that it's okay to ask for help!

When You Might Go Home

The decision about when you can leave the hospital after a liver transplant is based on how well you're healing and how ready you are to manage your recovery at home. For most patients, discharge happens about 1 to 2 weeks after surgery.

However, everyone recovers at their own pace, so your timeline might be a little different. Your medical team will carefully monitor your progress and make sure you're ready before giving you the green light to go home.

How Doctors Determine Readiness for Discharge

Before sending you home, your doctors will look at several important factors to make sure it's safe. Here are the main things they'll check:

1. ***Stable Liver Function***: Blood tests will show whether your new liver is working as expected. These tests help the doctors see if your body is accepting the new organ and how it's handling the changes.

2. ***Mobility and Independence***: You'll need to show that you can move around enough for basic daily activities, like getting out of bed, walking to the bathroom, or sitting up to eat. While you won't need to be fully mobile yet, being able to do small tasks is an important sign that you're recovering.
3. ***Wound Healing***: The surgical site will be closely monitored to make sure it's healing properly. Doctors will check for signs of infection, such as redness, swelling, or drainage. They'll also see if you or your caregiver can handle any wound care that's needed at home.
4. ***Medication Management***: You and your caregiver will need to feel confident about managing your medications at home. This includes knowing what to take, when to take it, and how to handle storage or possible side effects. The medical team will help you practice and answer any questions so that you're fully prepared.

The Role of Follow-Up Appointments

Leaving the hospital is just the beginning of your recovery. Regular follow-up visits are a key part of ensuring your long-term health after the transplant. These appointments are especially frequent in the first several weeks after surgery, allowing your doctors to monitor your progress closely.

- ***Liver Monitoring***: At each visit, your doctor will check how well your liver is working. Blood tests will be used to catch any potential issues early.
- ***Adjusting Medications***: Follow-ups are also a time to fine-tune your medications. Your doctors may adjust doses or change prescriptions based on how your body is responding.
- ***Catching Complications Early***: Any warning signs of infection, rejection, or other complications can often be addressed quickly during these appointments. Early action helps prevent problems from becoming more serious.

Going home is an exciting step, but it's normal to feel a bit nervous about managing things outside of the hospital. Remember, your medical team will continue to support you through follow-ups and is just a phone call away if you have questions or concerns. Take things one day at a time and lean on your caregiver for help during this period.

The Caregiver's Role After Discharge

Caregivers play a vital role in a liver transplant patient's recovery, especially in the early weeks at home. This section offers practical tips to help make the recovery process easier for both the patient and caregiver.

1. ***Managing Medications***: One of the most important tasks for a caregiver is helping the patient stick to their

medication schedule, especially for anti-rejection medications. These drugs are critical because they prevent the patient's immune system from attacking the new liver.

What to Do:

- Make sure medications are taken at the right time and in the correct dose every day.
- Use tools like a pill organizer, phone alarms, or charts to stay on track and avoid missed doses.
- If a medication runs low or side effects appear, contact the transplant team immediately for guidance.

2. ***Monitoring Recovery***: Part of your role is to keep an eye on the patient's health and be aware of changes that might signal a problem.

What to Watch for:

- Look for signs like jaundice (yellowing of the skin), fever, swelling, or unusual pain. These could indicate a complication and require prompt attention.
- Keep a record of the patient's daily weight, temperature, and any symptoms they experience. Bring this information to follow-up appointments so the medical team can better assess progress.

3. ***Encouraging Healthy Habits***: Supporting the patient with healthy routines is a big part of helping them heal. Recovery doesn't stop at medical care; everyday habits also make a big difference.

   How You Can Help:

   - Assist with meal preparation to ensure the patient eats balanced, nutritious meals that promote healing and liver health.
   - Encourage hydration by helping them drink enough water each day.
   - Motivate the patient to go for short walks or do light physical activities as recommended by the medical team. This improves circulation and strength.
   - Create a peaceful home environment that gives the patient plenty of rest and reduces stress. Small things like keeping the house quiet and organized can have a big impact.

4. ***Helping with Appointments and Organization***: There will be frequent doctor visits in the weeks after discharge, and staying organized is key to staying on top of the recovery process.

   What to Do:

   - Drive the patient to follow-up appointments if they can't go alone.

- Keep important documents, prescriptions, and instructions from the medical team all in one place for easy access.
- Help plan and manage the schedule for appointments, tests, and medication refills.

5. ***Taking Care of Yourself***: It's natural to focus most of your attention on the patient, but your well-being matters just as much. Being a caregiver can be physically and emotionally tiring, so prioritizing your health will help you provide the best possible care.

<u>Self-Care Tips:</u>

- Take Breaks: Don't hesitate to ask friends or family members to step in when you need time to recharge. Even short breaks can help you feel more balanced.
- Eat Well and Rest: Make sure you're eating nutritious meals, staying hydrated, and getting a good night's sleep.
- Build a Support Network: Join a caregiver support group to share experiences and gain emotional support. Talking to others in similar roles can help you feel less isolated.
- Address Your Own Health Needs: Keep up with your own doctor appointments and don't ignore any health concerns you might have.

Recovery is a team effort between the patient, caregiver, and medical team. Caregivers provide support and encouragement, while the transplant team offers guidance. Though the journey may have challenges, it leads to healing and a healthier, more fulfilling life.

Your First 30 Days Post-Transplant

The first month after a liver transplant is full of change, adjustment, and recovery. While it's an exciting time because you've been given a new chance at life, it can also feel overwhelming. Regular routines will look different, and there's much to learn about managing your health and preventing complications.

This chapter will help you understand how to ease into this next stage, so you feel prepared, supported, and informed.

Building New Routines

Adapting to post-transplant life starts with creating a structure that works for your recovery. It's important to take things one day at a time, focusing on healing and following your medical team's guidance.

- *Listen to Your Body*: After surgery, fatigue is normal. Your body needs time to adjust to the new liver and recover from the procedure. Rest when you need to, and don't push yourself too hard. Balance relaxation

with light activities, such as walking around the house, as recommended by your doctors.
- ***Stay Organized***: Create a daily schedule or checklist to keep track of medications, follow-up appointments, and other tasks. Tools like calendars or medication reminder apps can be helpful. Caregivers can also step in to help you stay on top of these commitments.
- ***Practice Good Hygiene***: To minimize the risk of infections, proper hygiene is critical. Wash your hands frequently, shower daily, and follow wound care instructions for your surgical incision.
- ***Monitor Progress***: Track your weight, blood pressure, and temperature daily, or as instructed by your transplant team. Noticing changes early can help identify issues before they escalate.

Recovering after a liver transplant takes time, patience, and a structured routine. By listening to your body, staying organized, and following medical advice, you can support your healing journey and build a healthier future.

Medication Management: What You Need to Know

One of the most vital parts of post-transplant care is managing your medications. These drugs help your body accept the new liver and prevent complications, but they come with responsibilities.

- ***Anti-Rejection Medications***: These are called immunosuppressants, and they make sure your immune system doesn't attack and reject the new liver. You'll likely need to take them for life, though your doctor may adjust the dosage over time. Make sure to take these exactly as prescribed and never skip a dose.
- ***Additional Medicines***: Beyond anti-rejection drugs, you may also need medicines to manage side effects, protect against infections, or treat other health conditions. Your care team will explain the purpose of each medication.
- ***Sticking to a Routine***: Setting reminders on your phone, using a pill organizer, or asking a caregiver for help can ensure you never miss a dose. Create a habit of taking your medication at the same times each day.
- ***Communicating with Your Medical Team***: If you experience side effects, such as nausea or unusual fatigue, inform your doctors. Some medications may need adjustments based on how your body responds.

Proper medication management is essential for a successful recovery and long-term health after a liver transplant. Stay consistent, communicate with your care team, and follow their guidance to ensure the best outcomes.

Signs Something May Be Wrong (and What to Do)

It's crucial to know what warning signs to watch for so you can act quickly if something doesn't feel right. Early action can prevent serious complications.

- *Rejection of the Liver*: Rejection can happen if your body's immune system sees the new liver as foreign, even with medications. Symptoms may include fever, fatigue, dark urine, jaundice (yellowing of the skin or eyes), or abdominal pain. Contact your transplant team immediately if you notice these signs.
- *Signs of Infection*: Because you're on immunosuppressants, your body's ability to fight infections is lower. Look out for fever, chills, persistent cough, redness or swelling around the incision site, or any unusual pain. Cleanliness and regular checkups help reduce infection risks.
- *Medication Side Effects*: Some people might experience tremors, weight gain, or swelling as side effects of the medications. Mention these to your doctor right away; they may adjust your treatment.
- *When to Call for Help*: If you experience severe symptoms, like trouble breathing, confusion, or extreme swelling in your legs or abdomen, go to an emergency room or contact your medical team without delay.

Recognizing warning signs early is key to staying healthy after a liver transplant. Always communicate any concerns with your medical team to ensure timely care and prevent complications.

Setting Up a Safe and Supportive Home Environment

The recovery process starts at the hospital, but much of it will continue at home. A well-prepared, supportive environment can make those early weeks smoother for both patients and caregivers.

- *Cleanliness Is Key*: Keep frequently touched surfaces, such as doorknobs and counters, clean. Avoid exposure to sick individuals or crowded places to reduce infection risk.
- *Create Comfortable Spaces*: Set up a cozy recovery area with easy access to necessities, like pillows, blankets, water, and medications. This might include having a recliner or bed in a quiet area where you can rest undisturbed.
- *Healthy Eating at Home*: Your nutrition needs will change post-transplant. A balanced diet with low salt and limited fatty foods may help recovery (more details are covered in Chapter 7). Stock up on easy-to-prepare meals and fresh produce.

- ***Support from Caregivers***: Whether it's a family member, friend, or hired help, having someone who can assist with errands, meals, or simply emotional encouragement is invaluable during this time. They'll also play a key role in helping track your medications, appointments, and symptoms.
- ***Stay Connected to Your Medical Team***: Even while at home, maintain close communication with your transplant team. Virtual check-ins can provide extra support in between in-person visits.

The first 30 days after a liver transplant will come with its challenges, but it's also a time to establish habits and routines that will set you up for success in the months and years to come. By staying organized, following medical advice, and prioritizing rest and hygiene, you'll set a strong foundation for your recovery. Caregivers play a crucial role in this period too, so lean on their support whenever needed.

Nutrition & Lifestyle for Liver Health

Maintaining a healthy diet and lifestyle is essential after a liver transplant to protect your new liver and support overall recovery. This chapter provides practical advice on eating well, staying active, managing stress, and getting enough rest during this critical time.

What to Eat and Avoid Post-Transplant

Your diet plays a key role in healing and keeping your liver healthy. Following dietary guidelines can help your body recover and prevent complications.

Foods to Include:

- *High-Protein Foods*: Promote healing and tissue repair with lean meats, eggs, beans, and low-fat dairy products.
- *Whole Grains*: Choose fiber-rich options like brown rice, quinoa, or whole wheat bread to support digestion.

- ***Fruits and Vegetables***: Aim for a variety of colorful produce to get essential vitamins, minerals, and antioxidants.
- ***Healthy Fats***: Incorporate moderate amounts of olive oil, avocados, nuts, and seeds for heart and liver health.
- ***Hydration***: Stay hydrated by drinking water throughout the day. Herbal teas or broths are also good options without added sugars.

Foods to Avoid:

- ***High-Sodium Foods***: Excess salt can cause fluid retention. Skip processed foods, canned soups, and salty snacks.
- ***Raw or Undercooked Foods***: Avoid sushi, raw oysters, or uncooked eggs to reduce the risk of infections.
- ***Alcohol***: Completely avoid alcohol, as it can damage your new liver.
- ***Sugary and Fatty Foods***: Limit sodas, candy, fast food, and fried items to avoid putting extra strain on your body.
- ***Grapefruit***: It interferes with some medications, particularly immunosuppressants.

Portion Control and Balance:

- Eat smaller, more frequent meals if large meals feel overwhelming.

- Balance your plate with protein, veggies, and whole grains at each meal.

Easy Meal Ideas and Grocery Tips

Creating nutritious meals doesn't have to be complicated. Here are suggestions for balanced meals and tips to simplify grocery shopping:

Meal Ideas:

1. ***Breakfast***: Scrambled eggs with spinach and whole-grain toast, plus a slice of melon.
2. ***Lunch***: Grilled chicken salad with mixed greens, cucumbers, and a light olive oil vinaigrette.
3. ***Dinner***: Baked salmon with quinoa and steamed broccoli.
4. ***Snacks***: Low-fat yogurt with a handful of berries, or carrot sticks with hummus.

Grocery Tips:

- ***Plan Ahead***: Write a meal plan for the week and make a shopping list based on it.
- ***Stick to the Perimeter***: Focus on fresh produce, dairy, and lean proteins, which are typically found around the outer edges of grocery stores.
- ***Read Labels***: Look for low-sodium and low-sugar options when buying packaged items.

- ***Freeze Extras***: Prepare meals in advance and freeze portions to save time and effort on busier days.

Simple, home-cooked meals can help you control ingredients and stay on track with your dietary needs.

Staying Active Without Overdoing It

Physical activity helps maintain liver health, manage weight, and improve overall fitness, but it's important to ease into exercise after surgery.

Light Exercises to Start With:

- ***Walking***: Short, gentle walks around your home or neighborhood are a great start. Gradually aim for 10–20 minutes at a time.
- ***Stretching***: Gentle yoga or light stretches improve flexibility and prevent stiffness.
- ***Chair Exercises***: Simple seated movements can help if standing for long periods is difficult.

Tips for Exercising Safely:

1. ***Listen to Your Body***: Stop immediately if you feel pain or dizziness.
2. ***Follow Doctor's Guidelines***: Get approval from your transplant team before starting any exercise program.
3. ***Gradual Progression***: Increase your activity levels steadily and avoid pushing yourself too soon.

4. ***Stay Hydrated***: Drink water before, during, and after exercising.

Many patients find that incorporating light movement into their daily routine improves energy levels and mood over time.

Importance of Sleep and Stress Management

Quality sleep and low stress levels are just as vital as diet and exercise in supporting liver health and recovery.

Tips for Improving Sleep:

- ***Create a Restful Environment***: Keep your bedroom dark, quiet, and cool.
- ***Set a Routine***: Go to bed and wake up at the same time each day, even on weekends.
- ***Limit Screen Time***: Avoid screens (phones, TVs, laptops) at least an hour before bed to improve sleep quality.
- ***Relax Before Bed***: Incorporate calming rituals like reading, gentle stretching, or listening to soothing music.

Managing Stress:

Stress can negatively affect your immune system and overall health. Try these techniques:

1. ***Mindfulness or Meditation***: Spend 5–10 minutes focusing on deep breathing or a simple guided meditation.
2. ***Journaling***: Writing down your thoughts and feelings can help relieve anxiety.
3. ***Support Groups***: Connecting with others who've had a liver transplant can provide emotional support and helpful advice.
4. ***Talk to Someone***: Don't hesitate to share your worries and fears with close family, friends, or a therapist.

Balancing sleep and stress management creates a strong foundation for recovery and overall well-being. Adopting liver-friendly nutrition and lifestyle habits can help you protect your transplant and feel your best.

Focus on making small, positive changes every day, and don't hesitate to reach out for support when you need it. With patience and dedication, these healthy habits will form a routine that supports your long-term health and happiness.

Long-Term Wellness and Support

A liver transplant is just the beginning of a lifelong commitment to prioritizing health and wellness. By staying proactive, you can maintain your new liver's health and build a thriving, balanced life. This chapter focuses on the critical elements of long-term care, from medical follow-ups to emotional and practical support.

Follow-Up Appointments and Lab Tests

Regular follow-ups are essential to ensuring your transplant continues to function well and to catch any problems early. These appointments help your healthcare team monitor your liver and overall health.

What to Expect During Follow-Ups:

1. *Physical Exam*: Your doctor will assess your general health and look for any signs of complications.
2. *Lab Tests*: Routine bloodwork checks liver function, medication levels, and signs of rejection or infection. Common tests include liver enzyme panels, bilirubin levels, and kidney function checks.

3. ***Imaging Tests***: Occasionally, scans like ultrasounds or MRIs may be ordered to get a detailed look at the liver if concerns arise.

Frequency of Follow-Ups:
- During the first year, follow-up visits often occur monthly or even weekly.
- Over time, they may decrease to every 3-6 months, depending on your progress and individual needs.
- Always attend these appointments, even if you feel great, to stay on top of your health.

Staying on Track with Your Medication

After a transplant, your medications are essential. They prevent rejection of your new liver and address other related health concerns. But keeping up with them can feel like a lot to manage.

- ***Building a Routine***: Take your medication at the same time(s) daily to develop a habit. Linking doses to a regular part of your schedule, like meals, can help. If you're forgetful, set phone alarms or use a smart pill dispenser that provides reminders.
- ***Avoiding Complications***: Skipping doses, altering your medication schedule, or stopping treatment on your own can be dangerous. If side effects occur, they need to be handled by your doctor, not by adjusting the

prescription yourself. Always consult your transplant team before making changes.
- **Communicating with Your Care Team**: Your medical team is your best resource for any medication-related questions or issues. Keep their contact information handy so you can reach them quickly if needed.
- **For Caregivers**: If you're helping someone stay on track, create tools like visual medication charts, pill organizers, or reminder alerts to simplify this daily responsibility.

Staying on top of your medication after a transplant is crucial for your health and recovery. With a solid routine, open communication with your care team, and helpful tools, you can manage your medication effectively and avoid complications.

How to Talk to Your Employer or Insurance

Navigating work and insurance post-transplant can feel complicated, but open communication and preparation can make it less stressful.

Talking to Your Employer:
- **Be Honest, But Selective**: Share only what's necessary about your health and any accommodations you might need, such as flexible hours for appointments or reduced workloads during recovery periods.

- ***Ask for Written Accommodations***: If your job involves physical labor, discuss options like light-duty roles or extended medical leave.
- ***Provide Documentation***: A note from your doctor explaining your condition and needs can help secure reasonable accommodations under workplace policies or laws like the ADA (Americans with Disabilities Act).

Navigating Insurance:

- ***Understand Your Coverage***: Review your insurance policy to understand what it covers, including medications, lab work, and follow-ups.
- ***Advocate for Yourself***: Contact your insurer about pre-approvals or appeals for denied claims, if necessary.
- ***Seek Financial Assistance***: Many organizations offer financial support for transplant-related expenses. Social workers at your transplant center can provide helpful resources.

By staying informed and advocating for your needs, you can navigate work and insurance challenges more confidently after a transplant. Remember, open communication and proper preparation are key to ensuring a smoother recovery and support system.

Joining Support Groups for Patients or Caregivers

The transplant process can be overwhelming for both patients and their caregivers. Connecting with support groups can provide emotional reassurance, practical advice, and a sense of community.

Benefits of Support Groups:

1. ***Shared Experiences***: Hearing from others who've been through similar situations can validate your feelings and give you a new perspective.
2. ***Advice and Tips***: Members often share how they've navigated challenges like medication routines, side effects, or unexpected setbacks.
3. ***Caregiver Support***: Caregivers also benefit from hearing the experiences of others, learning how to balance their role, and prioritizing their own well-being.

Finding Support Groups:

- ***Local Groups***: Hospitals, community centers, or transplant clinics may host in-person meetings.
- ***Online Communities***: Platforms like Facebook or forums offer virtual spaces where you can connect with others worldwide.

- ***Professional Guidance***: Social workers or transplant coordinators can recommend trustworthy groups tailored for your needs.

Life after a transplant comes with its challenges, but it also offers opportunities for growth and health. By keeping up with checkups, staying consistent with medications, and reaching out for support when needed, you can build a fulfilling future.

Conclusion

Thank you for taking the time to read this guide on liver transplants. By finishing it, you've equipped yourself with vital knowledge that can help you or your loved one face this life-changing procedure with confidence. Whether you're a patient or a caregiver, your decision to be informed is a powerful first step on the path to recovery.

A liver transplant is no small undertaking. It's a life-saving surgery that offers hope, renewed health, and a brighter future for patients. But just as important as the surgery itself is the ongoing care and commitment it takes to protect this second chance at life. Throughout this guide, we've explored everything from understanding liver disease to preparing for surgery, recovery, and long-term wellness. It's a lot to take in, but remember, you're not alone. You're surrounded by medical professionals, caregivers, and support networks who are ready to help you each step of the way.

This process may feel overwhelming at times, but know that it's okay to take things one step at a time. You don't have to have all the answers or figure everything out in one day.

Every small milestone, whether it's completing a follow-up appointment or taking your first post-surgery walk, is a victory. Celebrate progress, no matter how small, and trust the process. Healing takes time, patience, and perseverance.

If you're a caregiver, remember that your role is absolutely essential. Your support can make a world of difference to the patient as they heal not just physically, but emotionally too. But don't forget to care for yourself as well. Your well-being is just as important and allows you to continue being a source of strength and positivity.

One of the most powerful tools on this transplant journey is connection. Don't hesitate to lean on your transplant team, reach out to support groups, or ask for help from loved ones. Sharing experiences, asking questions, and seeking guidance can reduce stress and remind you that you're part of a community that genuinely cares about your success.

Most importantly, stay hopeful. A liver transplant represents a new chapter, one where better health and a higher quality of life are possible. Reflect on your reasons for taking this step, whether it's to live longer, enjoy more time with family, or regain the energy to pursue what you love. Keep those motivations close to your heart when things feel tough.

This is more than just a medical procedure—it's a transformation, an opportunity to reclaim your life. You're stronger than you think, and every challenge you face is another step toward healing and renewal. With determination, support, and the guidance of your transplant team, you can overcome this hurdle and thrive in your new phase of life.

FAQs

Who qualifies for a liver transplant?

A liver transplant is considered for individuals with severe liver damage or failure who cannot be treated through other methods. Common conditions include cirrhosis, hepatitis, acute liver failure, or congenital issues like biliary atresia. Your eligibility will depend on factors like overall health, MELD score, and readiness for surgery, which will be assessed by your transplant team.

What is a MELD score, and why is it important?

The MELD score (Model for End-Stage Liver Disease) helps prioritize patients on the transplant waiting list. It's calculated using lab results to measure how severe your liver disease is. A higher MELD score indicates a greater need for a transplant. Your doctor will explain your score and how it impacts your placement on the waiting list.

How long does it take to recover from a liver transplant?

Recovery is different for everyone but typically takes several months. Most patients stay in the hospital for 1–2 weeks post-surgery. During the first 30 days, you'll focus on healing, managing medications, and adjusting to your new routine. Full recovery, including regaining strength and returning to normal activities, can take 6–12 months.

What medications will I need to take after the transplant?

After a transplant, you'll take anti-rejection medications (immunosuppressants) to prevent your body from rejecting the new liver. You'll also need additional medications to protect against infections and manage side effects. It's important to take these as prescribed for the rest of your life to ensure the success of your transplant.

What lifestyle changes are needed after a liver transplant?

Post-transplant, a healthy lifestyle is essential to protect your new liver. You'll need to eat a balanced diet, avoid alcohol entirely, stay active without overdoing it, and prioritize sleep and stress management. Hygiene is also crucial to reduce the risk of infections, as your immune system will be suppressed due to medication.

What are the signs of liver rejection or complications?

Rejection or complications may present with symptoms like fever, jaundice (yellowing of the skin or eyes), dark urine, abdominal pain, swelling, or fatigue. Promptly report any of these signs to your transplant team. Regular follow-ups and bloodwork will also help monitor for any issues.

How can caregivers support someone during recovery?

Caregivers play a key role in helping with medication management, preparing meals, encouraging light activity, and attending follow-up appointments. They should also monitor for warning signs of complications. Just as importantly, caregivers need to prioritize their own physical and emotional well-being to provide sustainable support.

References and Helpful Links

Liver transplant - Mayo Clinic. (n.d.). https://www.mayoclinic.org/tests-procedures/liver-transplant/about/pac-20384842

Types of Liver Diseases that Lead to Transplantation. (n.d.). UPMC Children's Hospital of Pittsburgh. https://www.chp.edu/our-services/transplant/liver/liver-transplant-necessary/liver-diseases-transplant

Lifestyle changes after LIver transplantation. (n.d.). UPMC Children's Hospital of Pittsburgh. https://www.chp.edu/our-services/transplant/liver/recovery/coping/lifestyle-changes-after-liver-transplant#:~:text=Maintain%20general%20health%20through%20proper,to%20prevent%20infection%2C%20as%20prescribed.

Life after a liver transplant. (2022, June 23). Temple Health. https://www.templehealth.org/about/blog/life-after-liver-transplant

Pre-Liver Transplant Evaluation & Tests | UPMC. (n.d.). UPMC | Life Changing Medicine. https://www.upmc.com/services/transplant/liver/process/before#:~:text=Your%20pre%2Dliver%20transplant%20assessment%20will%20last%20one%20week.,transplant%20is%20right%20for%20you.

Food safety after a liver transplant - British Liver Trust. (2025, March 27). British Liver Trust. https://britishlivertrust.org.uk/information-and-support/living-with-a-liver-condition/food-safety-after-a-liver-transplant/

Understanding MELD score for liver transplant | UPMC. (n.d.). UPMC | Life Changing Medicine. https://www.upmc.com/services/transplant/liver/process/waiting-list/meld-score

www.ingramcontent.com/pod-product-compliance
Lightning Source LLC
LaVergne TN
LVHW012033060526
838201LV00061B/4584